Fertile Pathways

CNS

Fertile Pathways

Helping You Successfully Navigate IVF Stimulation with CNS Storks

Complete
Nurturing
Solutions
Childress Nursing Services

www.ChildressNursing.com

CNS

CHILDRESS PUBLISHING
P.O. Box 2031
Renton, WA 98056

www.ChildressNursing.com

ISBN 978-0-9979977-5-0

Complete Nurturing Solutions
Childress Nursing Services

Childress Nursing Services
SocioMaternal home health:
from preconception to post-delivery
Phone: 206-310-5101
Email: Contact@ChildressNursing.com
Website: www.ChildressNursing.com

Childress Nursing Services

Special Delivery For

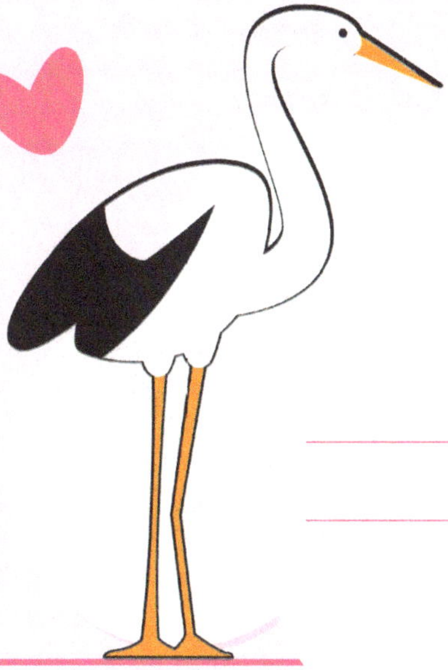

"Clients Corner"

There are no real words to express how thankful we are for all your help. You have really made this process so much easier for us and we really want you to know how not only you are a great nurse but an amazing genuine person. Your personality alone and presence brightens a room and changes our mood. Thanks so so much for everything.

♡

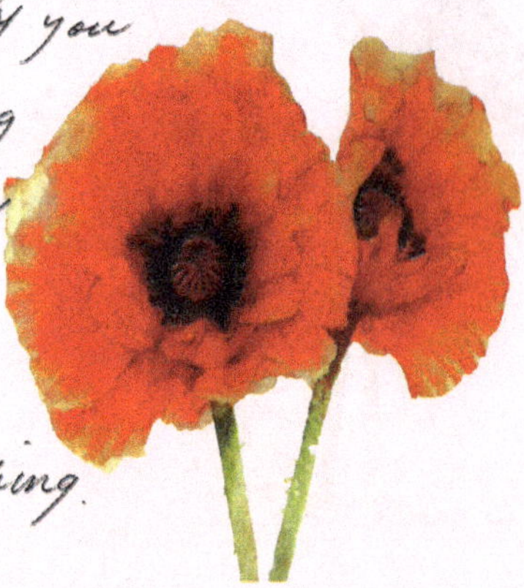

Table of Contents

My RECOMMENDED ITEM LIST

01	Childress Nursing Services' fertility workbook	☐
02	Arnicare gel (1 to 2 tubes)	☐
03	Hydrocortisone cream (1 tube) - optional	☐
04	Cold ice packs (2 packs)	☐
05	Heating pad (XL) - if transferring	☐
06	Gauze pads (2x2 - ideal size)	☐
07	Bandages (circle) - for abdominal injections	☐
08	Bandages (rectangle) - for IM injections	☐
09	Alcohol pads (if not included with meds)	☐

OPTIONAL MEDICATIONS:
Tylenol OTC, Benadryl OTC

**NO NSAIDS (ex. Ibuprofen, Naproxen)*

OTHER ITEMS:

My NOTES

Date:

My CNS HEALTH ASSESSMENTS

Vital Signs & Measurements

Date of *Initial* Assessment: ________________ Notes: ______________ Initial weight: _____ (lbs)

Blood Pressure	Temp (F)	Pulse (bpm)	Respirations	SpO2 (%)	Bowel Sounds	Abdominal Girth

Date of Assessment: ____________________________ Notes: ____________________________

Blood Pressure	Temp (F)	Pulse (bpm)	Respirations	SpO2 (%)	Bowel Sounds	Abdominal Girth

Date of Assessment: ____________________________ Notes: ____________________________

Blood Pressure	Temp (F)	Pulse (bpm)	Respirations	SpO2 (%)	Bowel Sounds	Abdominal Girth

Date of Assessment: ____________________________ Notes: ____________________________

Blood Pressure	Temp (F)	Pulse (bpm)	Respirations	SpO2 (%)	Bowel Sounds	Abdominal Girth

Date of Assessment: ____________________________ Notes: ____________________________

Blood Pressure	Temp (F)	Pulse (bpm)	Respirations	SpO2 (%)	Bowel Sounds	Abdominal Girth

My FERTILITY FOODS

Market:

SEAFOOD

POULTRY

DAIRY

VEGGIES/FRUITS

My ACTIVITIES

TO DO

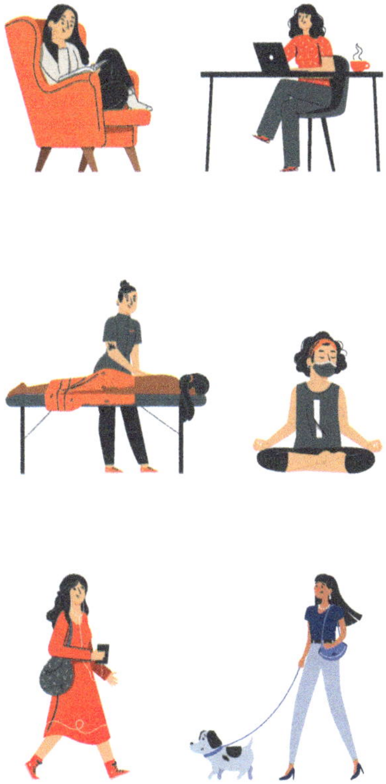

AVOID

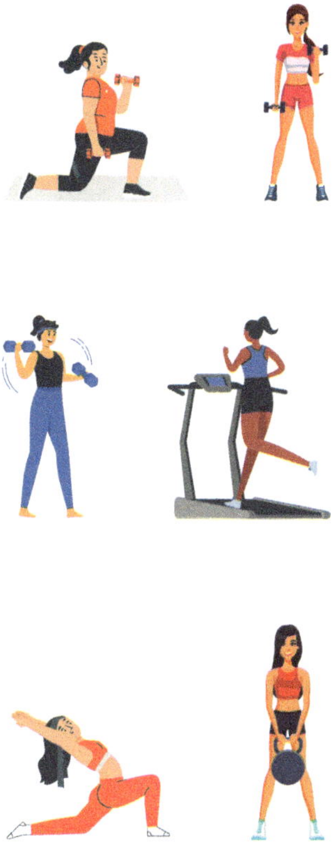

My MEDS

IVF STIMULATION MEDS OVERVIEW

Common Side Effects

Headache, abdominal ____________&____________, breast ________ /________, redness/slight bleeding/pain at the injection ______________________________

Common Med Names & Uses

Gonal-F

Contains follicle-stimulating hormone (FSH) and helps _____________ healthy ovaries to produce follicles.

Cetrotide

Blocks the release of lutenizing hormone (LH) resulting in preventing the eggs from being released ___________ and gives the eggs time to grow properly.

Trigger Shots

Given ___________ finishing your other fertility medications in the IVF stimulation phase to cause ovulation or the release of eggs from ovaries.

*Given exactly ______________ hours before egg retrieval.

- Human Chorionic Gonadotropin (HCG)
- Ovidrel
- Lupron

Menopur

contains follicle-stimulating hormone (FSH) and luteinizing hormone (LH) that helps healthy ovaries to make follicles. *___________________ sensation*

Omnitrope

Synthetic growth hormone that increases ___________ levels in body to stimulate ovulation, improves egg quality and helps with egg maturation.

Lupron

Prevents premature surge of LH before _____________.

My NOTES

Date:

"CLients Corner"

Dear

Thank you for your support through the IVF process. You are an angle and we are forever grateful.

At my baby shower I was going to give you this Glassy Baby "Celebrate" as a token of my appreciation to you in helping us create Life. I hope it brings you Joy for years. We Celebrated Nathaniel in style on May

We Send you love.

My CYCLE # ________

Start Date:

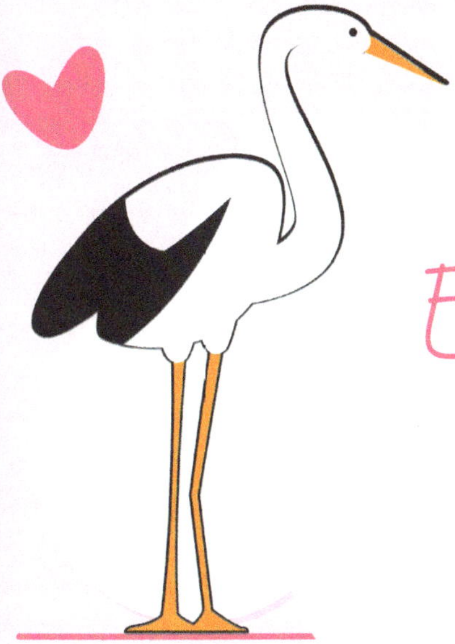

Enjoy The Process

My MED CHECKS

Date of *Initial* Med Check: ______________ Notes: ______________________________

Date	Med Name & Dosage	# of doses remaining	Earliest Reorder date	Storage after opening

Date	Med Name & Dosage	# of doses remaining	Earliest Reorder date	Storage after opening

Date	Med Name & Dosage	# of doses remaining	Earliest Reorder date	Storage after opening

Date	Med Name & Dosage	# of doses remaining	Earliest Reorder date	Storage after opening

Date	Med Name & Dosage	# of doses remaining	Earliest Reorder date	Storage after opening

Date	Med Name & Dosage	# of doses remaining	Earliest Reorder date	Storage after opening

Date	Med Name & Dosage	# of doses remaining	Earliest Reorder date	Storage after opening

★ Note: Meds generally expire within 28 days of piercing vial or by expiration date, whichever is sooner.

C N S

My IVF SCHEDULE

SUPPRESION CHECK:	STIM DAY 1	STIM DAY 2	STIM DAY 3	STIM DAY 4
BASELINE ULTRASOUND & BLOOD TEST	Start Stim Meds			
	PM Stim Meds: Gonal-F / FSH / Menopur / MiniHCG / Omnitrope			
Period day 1	AM Meds : If on Lupron protocol, continue Lupron AM			

STIM DAY 5	STIM DAY 6	STIM DAY 7	STIM DAY 8	STIM DAY 9
Day 5 or 6 1st AM Monitoring Appt.				Day 9 Appt.
PM Stim Meds: Gonal-F / FSH / Menopur / MiniHCG / Omnitrope				
AM Cetrotide / Ganirelix only once instructed to start *OR* continue Lupron				

STIM DAY 10	STIM DAY 11	STIM DAY 12	STIM DAY 13	STIM DAY 14
PM Stim Meds: Gonal-F / FSH / Menopur / MiniHCG / Omnitrope				
AM Cetrotide / Ganirelix *OR* continue Lupron				
90% chance of HCG PM Trigger			10% chance of HCG PM Trigger	
		90% chance of AM Egg Retrieval		

10% chance of AM Egg Retrieval

Fresh Embryo Transfer: 3 to 5 days post - Egg Retrieval *OR*
Frozen Embryo BIOPSY: 5 to 7 Days post-Egg Retrieval

IMPORTANT DATES / TIMES

(Email CNS office ASAP if outside your time window)

Clinic Monitoring Appointments

Day 5 / 6: ____ /____ /__________ Time: _______

Day 9: ____ /____ /___________ Time: _______

Day ___: ____ /____ /__________ Time: _______

Day ___: ____ /____ /__________ Time: _______

Day ___: ____ /____ /__________ Time: _______

Day ___: ____ /____ /__________ Time: _______

1st Cetrotide / Ganirelix shot

Date: ____ /____ /__________ Time: _______PM

Email CNS office ASAP with details!

Trigger Shot

Date: ____ /____ /__________ Time: _______PM

My APPOINTMENTS

DATE & TIME: ______________________ ______________________

APPOINTMENT TYPE: ______________________

☐ CONSULTATION	☐ CYCLE MONITORING	☐ EGG RETRIEVAL	☐ LABS
☐ PROCEDURE(S)	☐ ULTRASOUND	☐ FET/TRANSFER	☐ OTHER

QUESTIONS/CONCERNS BEFORE APPT/TOPICS DISCUSSED WITH CNS STORK:

____

____

INSTRUCTIONS/FOLLOW-UP/NOTES/EMAIL CNS OFFICE

____

____

BLOOD TEST

Date	Blood test type	Expected Normal Range(s)	My Results

FOLLICLE GROWTH

Date	Lining Thickness (mm)	Left Ovary		Right Ovary	
		#	Size	#	Size

My APPOINTMENTS

DATE & TIME: ______________________ ______________________

APPOINTMENT TYPE: ______________________

- ❒ CONSULTATION
- ❒ CYCLE MONITORING
- ❒ EGG RETRIEVAL
- ❒ LABS
- ❒ PROCEDURE(S)
- ❒ ULTRASOUND
- ❒ FET/TRANSFER
- ❒ OTHER

QUESTIONS/CONCERNS BEFORE APPT/TOPICS DISCUSSED WITH CNS STORK:

____

____

INSTRUCTIONS/FOLLOW-UP/NOTES/EMAIL CNS OFFICE

____

____

BLOOD TEST

Date	Blood test type	Expected Normal Range(s)	My Results

FOLLICLE GROWTH

Date	Lining Thickness (mm)	Left Ovary		Right Ovary	
		#	Size	#	Size

My APPOINTMENTS

DATE & TIME: ______________________ ______________________

APPOINTMENT TYPE: ____

- ❑ CONSULTATION
- ❑ CYCLE MONITORING
- ❑ EGG RETRIEVAL
- ❑ LABS
- ❑ PROCEDURE(S)
- ❑ ULTRASOUND
- ❑ FET/TRANSFER
- ❑ OTHER

QUESTIONS/CONCERNS BEFORE APPT/TOPICS DISCUSSED WITH CNS STORK:

INSTRUCTIONS/FOLLOW-UP/NOTES/EMAIL CNS OFFICE

BLOOD TEST

Date	Blood test type	Expected Normal Range(s)	My Results

FOLLICLE GROWTH

Date	Lining Thickness (mm)	Left Ovary		Right Ovary	
		#	Size	#	Size

My APPOINTMENTS

DATE & TIME: ______________________ ______________________

APPOINTMENT TYPE: ______________________

☐ CONSULTATION	☐ CYCLE MONITORING	☐ EGG RETRIEVAL	☐ LABS
☐ PROCEDURE(S)	☐ ULTRASOUND	☐ FET/TRANSFER	☐ OTHER

QUESTIONS/CONCERNS BEFORE APPT/TOPICS DISCUSSED WITH CNS STORK:

INSTRUCTIONS/FOLLOW-UP/NOTES/EMAIL CNS OFFICE

BLOOD TEST

Date	Blood test type	Expected Normal Range(s)	My Results

FOLLICLE GROWTH

Date	Lining Thickness (mm)	Left Ovary		Right Ovary	
		#	Size	#	Size

My APPOINTMENTS

DATE & TIME: ______________________ ______________________

APPOINTMENT TYPE: ______________________

☐ CONSULTATION	☐ CYCLE MONITORING	☐ EGG RETRIEVAL	☐ LABS
☐ PROCEDURE(S)	☐ ULTRASOUND	☐ FET/TRANSFER	☐ OTHER

QUESTIONS/CONCERNS BEFORE APPT/TOPICS DISCUSSED WITH CNS STORK:

____

____

INSTRUCTIONS/FOLLOW-UP/NOTES/EMAIL CNS OFFICE

____

____

BLOOD TEST

Date	Blood test type	Expected Normal Range(s)	My Results

FOLLICLE GROWTH

Date	Lining Thickness (mm)	Left Ovary		Right Ovary	
		#	Size	#	Size

My APPOINTMENTS

DATE & TIME: ______________________ ______________________

APPOINTMENT TYPE: ______________________

❐ CONSULTATION	❐ CYCLE MONITORING	❐ EGG RETRIEVAL	❐ LABS
❐ PROCEDURE(S)	❐ ULTRASOUND	❐ FET/TRANSFER	❐ OTHER

QUESTIONS/CONCERNS BEFORE APPT/TOPICS DISCUSSED WITH CNS STORK:

INSTRUCTIONS/FOLLOW-UP/NOTES/EMAIL CNS OFFICE

BLOOD TEST

Date	Blood test type	Expected Normal Range(s)	My Results

FOLLICLE GROWTH

Date	Lining Thickness (mm)	Left Ovary		Right Ovary	
		#	Size	#	Size

My INJECTIONS

Care Period: ______________ to ______________

Date ____/_____/____________ Symptoms / Comments: ______________________________

Med Name & Dosage	Route	Site #	Stork Name

Date ____/_____/____________ Symptoms / Comments: ______________________________

Med Name & Dosage	Route	Site #	Stork Name

Date ____/_____/____________ Symptoms / Comments: ______________________________

Med Name & Dosage	Route	Site #	Stork Name

Date ____/_____/____________ Symptoms / Comments: ______________________________

Med Name & Dosage	Route	Site #	Stork Name

Date ____/_____/____________ Symptoms / Comments: ______________________________

Med Name & Dosage	Route	Site #	Stork Name

Date ____/_____/____________ Symptoms / Comments: ______________________________

Med Name & Dosage	Route	Site #	Stork Name

Date ____/_____/____________ Symptoms / Comments: ______________________________

Med Name & Dosage	Route	Site #	Stork Name

Date ____/_____/____________ Symptoms / Comments: ______________________________

Med Name & Dosage	Route	Site #	Stork Name

INJECTION SITES:

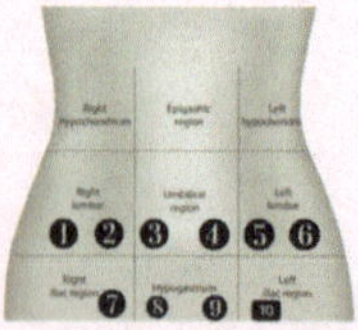

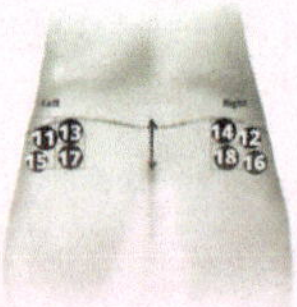

My INJECTIONS

Care Period: ______________ to ______________

Date ____ /_____ /____________ Symptoms / Comments: ______________________________

Med Name & Dosage	Route	Site #	Stork Name

Date ____ /_____ /____________ Symptoms / Comments: ______________________________

Med Name & Dosage	Route	Site #	Stork Name

Date ____ /_____ /____________ Symptoms / Comments: ______________________________

Med Name & Dosage	Route	Site #	Stork Name

Date ____ /_____ /____________ Symptoms / Comments: ______________________________

Med Name & Dosage	Route	Site #	Stork Name

Date ____ /_____ /____________ Symptoms / Comments: ______________________________

Med Name & Dosage	Route	Site #	Stork Name

Date ____ /_____ /____________ Symptoms / Comments: ______________________________

Med Name & Dosage	Route	Site #	Stork Name

Date ____ /_____ /____________ Symptoms / Comments: ______________________________

Med Name & Dosage	Route	Site #	Stork Name

Date ____ /_____ /____________ Symptoms / Comments: ______________________________

Med Name & Dosage	Route	Site #	Stork Name

INJECTION SITES:

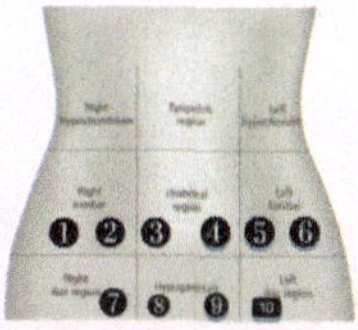

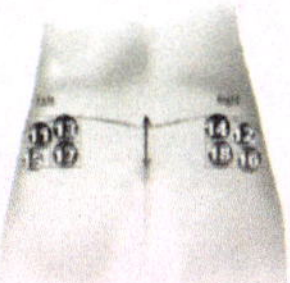

My INJECTIONS

Care Period: ______________ to ______________

Date ____ /_____ /____________ Symptoms / Comments: ______________________________

Med Name & Dosage	Route	Site #	Stork Name

Date ____ /_____ /____________ Symptoms / Comments: ______________________________

Med Name & Dosage	Route	Site #	Stork Name

Date ____ /_____ /____________ Symptoms / Comments: ______________________________

Med Name & Dosage	Route	Site #	Stork Name

Date ____ /_____ /____________ Symptoms / Comments: ______________________________

Med Name & Dosage	Route	Site #	Stork Name

Date ____ /_____ /____________ Symptoms / Comments: ______________________________

Med Name & Dosage	Route	Site #	Stork Name

Date ____ /_____ /____________ Symptoms / Comments: ______________________________

Med Name & Dosage	Route	Site #	Stork Name

Date ____ /_____ /____________ Symptoms / Comments: ______________________________

Med Name & Dosage	Route	Site #	Stork Name

Date ____ /_____ /____________ Symptoms / Comments: ______________________________

Med Name & Dosage	Route	Site #	Stork Name

INJECTION SITES:

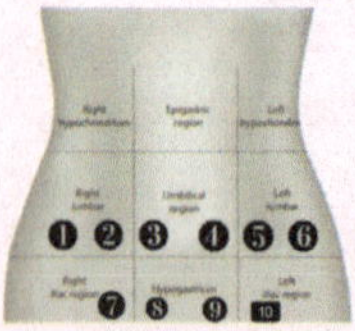

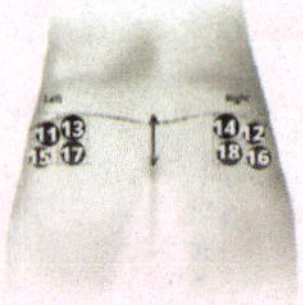

My INJECTIONS

Care Period: ______________ to ______________

Date ____ /____ /____________ Symptoms / Comments: ______________________________

Med Name & Dosage	Route	Site #	Stork Name

Date ____ /____ /____________ Symptoms / Comments: ______________________________

Med Name & Dosage	Route	Site #	Stork Name

Date ____ /____ /____________ Symptoms / Comments: ______________________________

Med Name & Dosage	Route	Site #	Stork Name

Date ____ /____ /____________ Symptoms / Comments: ______________________________

Med Name & Dosage	Route	Site #	Stork Name

Date ____ /____ /____________ Symptoms / Comments: ______________________________

Med Name & Dosage	Route	Site #	Stork Name

Date ____ /____ /____________ Symptoms / Comments: ______________________________

Med Name & Dosage	Route	Site #	Stork Name

Date ____ /____ /____________ Symptoms / Comments: ______________________________

Med Name & Dosage	Route	Site #	Stork Name

Date ____ /____ /____________ Symptoms / Comments: ______________________________

Med Name & Dosage	Route	Site #	Stork Name

INJECTION SITES:

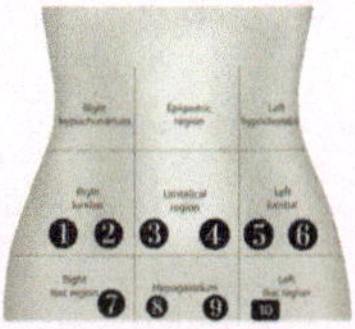

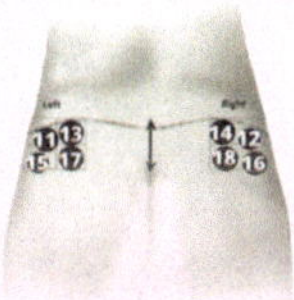

My INJECTIONS

Care Period: ______________ to ______________

Date ____/_____/____________ Symptoms / Comments: ______________________

Med Name & Dosage	Route	Site #	Stork Name

Date ____/_____/____________ Symptoms / Comments: ______________________

Med Name & Dosage	Route	Site #	Stork Name

Date ____/_____/____________ Symptoms / Comments: ______________________

Med Name & Dosage	Route	Site #	Stork Name

Date ____/_____/____________ Symptoms / Comments: ______________________

Med Name & Dosage	Route	Site #	Stork Name

Date ____/_____/____________ Symptoms / Comments: ______________________

Med Name & Dosage	Route	Site #	Stork Name

Date ____/_____/____________ Symptoms / Comments: ______________________

Med Name & Dosage	Route	Site #	Stork Name

Date ____/_____/____________ Symptoms / Comments: ______________________

Med Name & Dosage	Route	Site #	Stork Name

Date ____/_____/____________ Symptoms / Comments: ______________________

Med Name & Dosage	Route	Site #	Stork Name

INJECTION SITES:

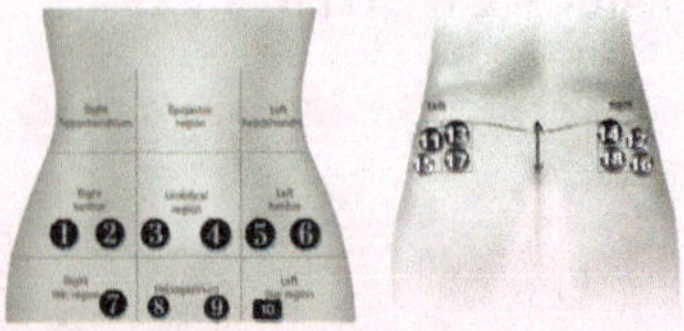

My INJECTIONS

Care Period: ______________ to ______________

Date ____ /_____ /____________ Symptoms / Comments: ______________________________

Med Name & Dosage	Route	Site #	Stork Name

Date ____ /_____ /____________ Symptoms / Comments: ______________________________

Med Name & Dosage	Route	Site #	Stork Name

Date ____ /_____ /____________ Symptoms / Comments: ______________________________

Med Name & Dosage	Route	Site #	Stork Name

Date ____ /_____ /____________ Symptoms / Comments: ______________________________

Med Name & Dosage	Route	Site #	Stork Name

Date ____ /_____ /____________ Symptoms / Comments: ______________________________

Med Name & Dosage	Route	Site #	Stork Name

Date ____ /_____ /____________ Symptoms / Comments: ______________________________

Med Name & Dosage	Route	Site #	Stork Name

Date ____ /_____ /____________ Symptoms / Comments: ______________________________

Med Name & Dosage	Route	Site #	Stork Name

Date ____ /_____ /____________ Symptoms / Comments: ______________________________

Med Name & Dosage	Route	Site #	Stork Name

INJECTION SITES:

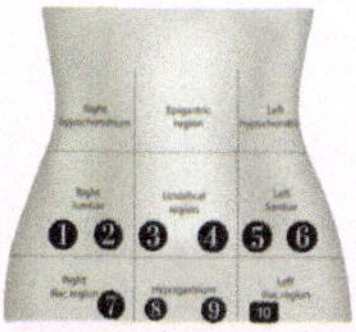

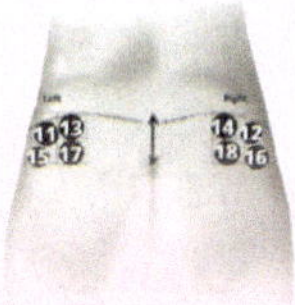

My NOTES

Date:

C N S

My EMBRYOS

Date: ______ /______ /__________ Follicles Retrieved: ______________________

Mature Follicles ________________ ICSI/PICSI: ______________________

Day	1	3	5	6	Blastocysts	Frozen	PGS Normal	PGS Abnormal
Qty								

pgt / pgs / pgd Results

Embryo #	Morphology	Embryo Result	Grade	Sex	Notes

Retrieval Day Check In

Doctor Name: ________________ Location: ______________________

My NOTES

Date:

"CLients Corner"

Thank you for everything & I could NOT do it without you & You have been a God sent & I appreciate yours great

GOODNESS

I will be LIKE YOURS in touch &

CAN'T BE EXPLAINED...

God Bless & just appreciated.

always know that you have been a true blessing in this process

Best,

-AND "Kids"

:)

Hugs
HB
etc

My CYCLE # ________

Start Date:

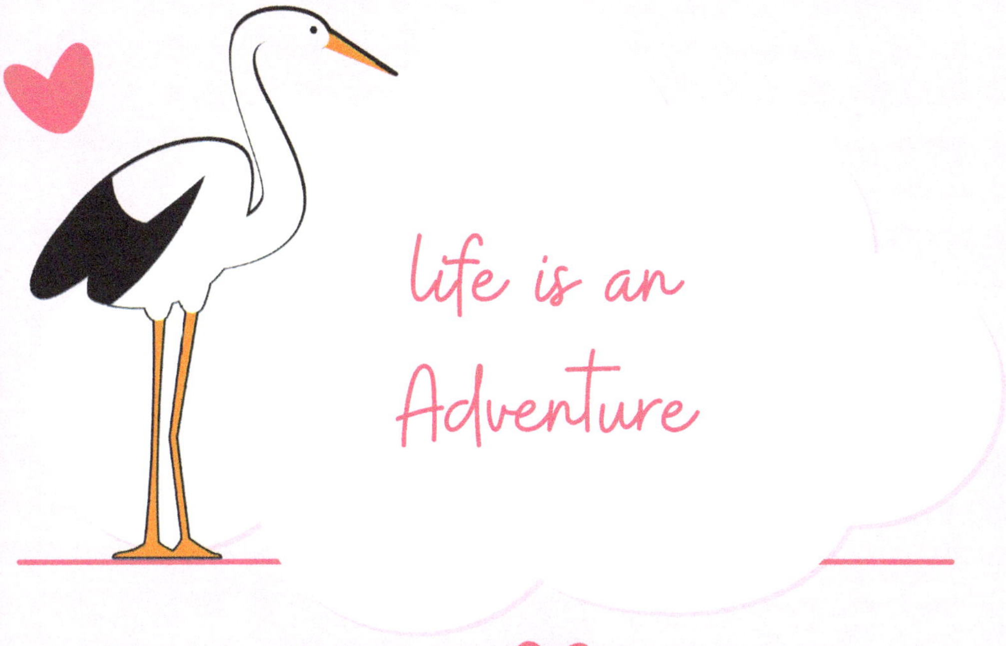

My MED CHECKS

Date of *Initial* Med Check: ____________________ Notes: ________________________________

Date	Med Name & Dosage	# of doses remaining	Earliest Reorder date	Storage after opening

Date	Med Name & Dosage	# of doses remaining	Earliest Reorder date	Storage after opening

Date	Med Name & Dosage	# of doses remaining	Earliest Reorder date	Storage after opening

Date	Med Name & Dosage	# of doses remaining	Earliest Reorder date	Storage after opening

Date	Med Name & Dosage	# of doses remaining	Earliest Reorder date	Storage after opening

Date	Med Name & Dosage	# of doses remaining	Earliest Reorder date	Storage after opening

Date	Med Name & Dosage	# of doses remaining	Earliest Reorder date	Storage after opening

★ Note: Meds generally expire within 28 days of piercing vial or by expiration date, whichever is sooner.

My IVF SCHEDULE

SUPPRESION CHECK:	STIM DAY 1	STIM DAY 2	STIM DAY 3	STIM DAY 4
BASELINE ULTRASOUND & BLOOD TEST	Start Stim Meds			
	PM Stim Meds: Gonal-F / FSH / Menopur / MiniHCG / Omnitrope			
Period day 1	AM Meds : If on Lupron protocol, continue Lupron AM			

STIM DAY 5	STIM DAY 6	STIM DAY 7	STIM DAY 8	STIM DAY 9
Day 5 or 6 1st AM Monitoring Appt.				Day 9 Appt.
PM Stim Meds: Gonal-F / FSH / Menopur / MiniHCG / Omnitrope				
AM Cetrotide / Ganirelix only once instructed to start *OR* continue Lupron				

STIM DAY 10	STIM DAY 11	STIM DAY 12	STIM DAY 13	STIM DAY 14
PM Stim Meds: Gonal-F / FSH / Menopur / MiniHCG / Omnitrope				
AM Cetrotide / Ganirelix *OR* continue Lupron				
90% chance of HCG PM Trigger			10% chance of HCG PM Trigger	
		90% chance of AM Egg Retrieval		

10% chance of AM Egg Retrieval

Fresh Embryo Transfer: 3 to 5 days post - Egg Retrieval *OR*
Frozen Embryo BIOPSY: 5 to 7 Days post-Egg Retrieval

IMPORTANT DATES / TIMES

(Email CNS office ASAP if outside your time window)

Clinic Monitoring Appointments

Day 5 / 6: ____ /____ /________ Time: ______

Day 9: ____ /____ /__________ Time: ______

Day ___: ____ /____ /________ Time: ______

Day ___: ____ /____ /________ Time: ______

Day ___: ____ /____ /________ Time: ______

Day ___: ____ /____ /________ Time: ______

1st Cetrotide / Ganirelix shot

Date: ____ /____ /__________ Time: ______PM

Email CNS office ASAP with details!

Trigger Shot

Date: ____ /____ /__________ Time: ______PM

My APPOINTMENTS

DATE & TIME: ______________________ ______________________

APPOINTMENT TYPE: ______________________

- ☐ CONSULTATION
- ☐ CYCLE MONITORING
- ☐ EGG RETRIEVAL
- ☐ LABS
- ☐ PROCEDURE(S)
- ☐ ULTRASOUND
- ☐ FET/TRANSFER
- ☐ OTHER

QUESTIONS/CONCERNS BEFORE APPT/TOPICS DISCUSSED WITH CNS STORK:

INSTRUCTIONS/FOLLOW-UP/NOTES/EMAIL CNS OFFICE

BLOOD TEST

Date	Blood test type	Expected Normal Range(s)	My Results

FOLLICLE GROWTH

Date	Lining Thickness (mm)	Left Ovary		Right Ovary	
		#	Size	#	Size

My APPOINTMENTS

DATE & TIME: ______________________ ______________________

APPOINTMENT TYPE: ______________________

- ❐ CONSULTATION
- ❐ CYCLE MONITORING
- ❐ EGG RETRIEVAL
- ❐ LABS
- ❐ PROCEDURE(S)
- ❐ ULTRASOUND
- ❐ FET/TRANSFER
- ❐ OTHER

QUESTIONS/CONCERNS BEFORE APPT/TOPICS DISCUSSED WITH CNS STORK:

INSTRUCTIONS/FOLLOW-UP/NOTES/EMAIL CNS OFFICE

BLOOD TEST

Date	Blood test type	Expected Normal Range(s)	My Results

FOLLICLE GROWTH

Date	Lining Thickness (mm)	Left Ovary		Right Ovary	
		#	Size	#	Size

My APPOINTMENTS

DATE & TIME: ______________________ ______________________

APPOINTMENT TYPE: ______________________

☐ CONSULTATION	☐ CYCLE MONITORING	☐ EGG RETRIEVAL	☐ LABS
☐ PROCEDURE(S)	☐ ULTRASOUND	☐ FET/TRANSFER	☐ OTHER

QUESTIONS/CONCERNS BEFORE APPT/TOPICS DISCUSSED WITH CNS STORK:

INSTRUCTIONS/FOLLOW-UP/NOTES/EMAIL CNS OFFICE

BLOOD TEST

Date	Blood test type	Expected Normal Range(s)	My Results

FOLLICLE GROWTH

Date	Lining Thickness (mm)	Left Ovary		Right Ovary	
		#	Size	#	Size

My APPOINTMENTS

DATE & TIME: ______________________________ ______________________________

APPOINTMENT TYPE: ______________________________

- ❑ CONSULTATION
- ❑ CYCLE MONITORING
- ❑ EGG RETRIEVAL
- ❑ LABS
- ❑ PROCEDURE(S)
- ❑ ULTRASOUND
- ❑ FET/TRANSFER
- ❑ OTHER

QUESTIONS/CONCERNS BEFORE APPT/TOPICS DISCUSSED WITH CNS STORK:

INSTRUCTIONS/FOLLOW-UP/NOTES/EMAIL CNS OFFICE

BLOOD TEST

Date	Blood test type	Expected Normal Range(s)	My Results

FOLLICLE GROWTH

Date	Lining Thickness (mm)	Left Ovary		Right Ovary	
		#	Size	#	Size

My APPOINTMENTS

DATE & TIME: ______________________ ______________________

APPOINTMENT TYPE: ______________________

- [ ] CONSULTATION
- [ ] CYCLE MONITORING
- [ ] EGG RETRIEVAL
- [ ] LABS
- [ ] PROCEDURE(S)
- [ ] ULTRASOUND
- [ ] FET/TRANSFER
- [ ] OTHER

QUESTIONS/CONCERNS BEFORE APPT/TOPICS DISCUSSED WITH CNS STORK:

INSTRUCTIONS/FOLLOW-UP/NOTES/EMAIL CNS OFFICE

BLOOD TEST

Date	Blood test type	Expected Normal Range(s)	My Results

FOLLICLE GROWTH

Date	Lining Thickness (mm)	Left Ovary		Right Ovary	
		#	Size	#	Size

My APPOINTMENTS

DATE & TIME: ____________________ ____________________

APPOINTMENT TYPE: ____

- ❒ CONSULTATION
- ❒ CYCLE MONITORING
- ❒ EGG RETRIEVAL
- ❒ LABS
- ❒ PROCEDURE(S)
- ❒ ULTRASOUND
- ❒ FET/TRANSFER
- ❒ OTHER

QUESTIONS/CONCERNS BEFORE APPT/TOPICS DISCUSSED WITH CNS STORK:

INSTRUCTIONS/FOLLOW-UP/NOTES/EMAIL CNS OFFICE

BLOOD TEST

Date	Blood test type	Expected Normal Range(s)	My Results

FOLLICLE GROWTH

Date	Lining Thickness (mm)	Left Ovary		Right Ovary	
		#	Size	#	Size

My INJECTIONS

Care Period: ______________ to ______________

Date ____ /_____ /____________ Symptoms / Comments: ______________________________

Med Name & Dosage	Route	Site #	Stork Name

Date ____ /_____ /____________ Symptoms / Comments: ______________________________

Med Name & Dosage	Route	Site #	Stork Name

Date ____ /_____ /____________ Symptoms / Comments: ______________________________

Med Name & Dosage	Route	Site #	Stork Name

Date ____ /_____ /____________ Symptoms / Comments: ______________________________

Med Name & Dosage	Route	Site #	Stork Name

Date ____ /_____ /____________ Symptoms / Comments: ______________________________

Med Name & Dosage	Route	Site #	Stork Name

Date ____ /_____ /____________ Symptoms / Comments: ______________________________

Med Name & Dosage	Route	Site #	Stork Name

Date ____ /_____ /____________ Symptoms / Comments: ______________________________

Med Name & Dosage	Route	Site #	Stork Name

Date ____ /_____ /____________ Symptoms / Comments: ______________________________

Med Name & Dosage	Route	Site #	Stork Name

INJECTION SITES:

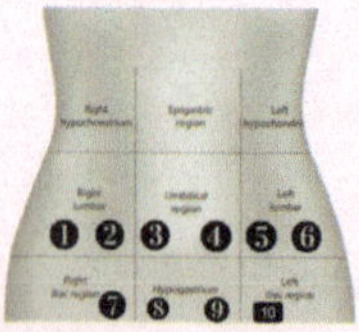

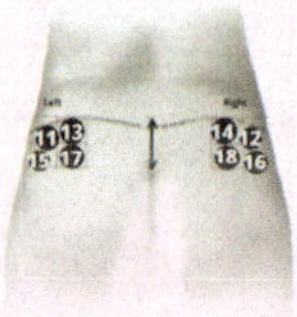

My INJECTIONS

Care Period: ______________ to ______________

Date ____ /_____ /____________ Symptoms / Comments: ______________________________

Med Name & Dosage	Route	Site #	Stork Name

Date ____ /_____ /____________ Symptoms / Comments: ______________________________

Med Name & Dosage	Route	Site #	Stork Name

Date ____ /_____ /____________ Symptoms / Comments: ______________________________

Med Name & Dosage	Route	Site #	Stork Name

Date ____ /_____ /____________ Symptoms / Comments: ______________________________

Med Name & Dosage	Route	Site #	Stork Name

Date ____ /_____ /____________ Symptoms / Comments: ______________________________

Med Name & Dosage	Route	Site #	Stork Name

Date ____ /_____ /____________ Symptoms / Comments: ______________________________

Med Name & Dosage	Route	Site #	Stork Name

Date ____ /_____ /____________ Symptoms / Comments: ______________________________

Med Name & Dosage	Route	Site #	Stork Name

Date ____ /_____ /____________ Symptoms / Comments: ______________________________

Med Name & Dosage	Route	Site #	Stork Name

INJECTION SITES:

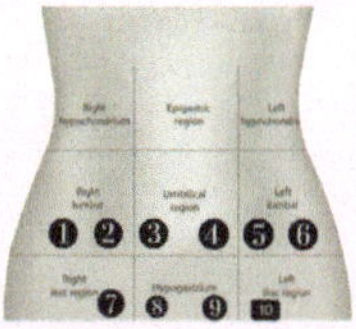

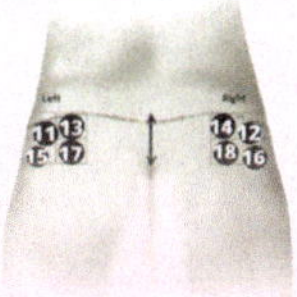

My INJECTIONS

Care Period: ________________ to ________________

Date ____/_____/_____________ Symptoms / Comments: ______________________________

Med Name & Dosage	Route	Site #	Stork Name

Date ____/_____/_____________ Symptoms / Comments: ______________________________

Med Name & Dosage	Route	Site #	Stork Name

Date ____/_____/_____________ Symptoms / Comments: ______________________________

Med Name & Dosage	Route	Site #	Stork Name

Date ____/_____/_____________ Symptoms / Comments: ______________________________

Med Name & Dosage	Route	Site #	Stork Name

Date ____/_____/_____________ Symptoms / Comments: ______________________________

Med Name & Dosage	Route	Site #	Stork Name

Date ____/_____/_____________ Symptoms / Comments: ______________________________

Med Name & Dosage	Route	Site #	Stork Name

Date ____/_____/_____________ Symptoms / Comments: ______________________________

Med Name & Dosage	Route	Site #	Stork Name

Date ____/_____/_____________ Symptoms / Comments: ______________________________

Med Name & Dosage	Route	Site #	Stork Name

INJECTION SITES:

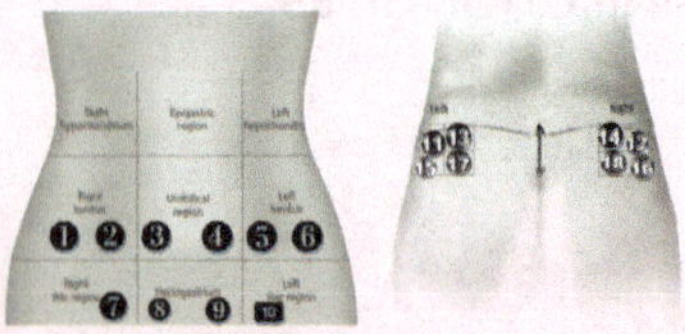

My INJECTIONS

Care Period: ______________ to ______________

Date ____ /_____ /____________ Symptoms / Comments: ______________________________

Med Name & Dosage	Route	Site #	Stork Name

Date ____ /_____ /____________ Symptoms / Comments: ______________________________

Med Name & Dosage	Route	Site #	Stork Name

Date ____ /_____ /____________ Symptoms / Comments: ______________________________

Med Name & Dosage	Route	Site #	Stork Name

Date ____ /_____ /____________ Symptoms / Comments: ______________________________

Med Name & Dosage	Route	Site #	Stork Name

Date ____ /_____ /____________ Symptoms / Comments: ______________________________

Med Name & Dosage	Route	Site #	Stork Name

Date ____ /_____ /____________ Symptoms / Comments: ______________________________

Med Name & Dosage	Route	Site #	Stork Name

Date ____ /_____ /____________ Symptoms / Comments: ______________________________

Med Name & Dosage	Route	Site #	Stork Name

Date ____ /_____ /____________ Symptoms / Comments: ______________________________

Med Name & Dosage	Route	Site #	Stork Name

INJECTION SITES:

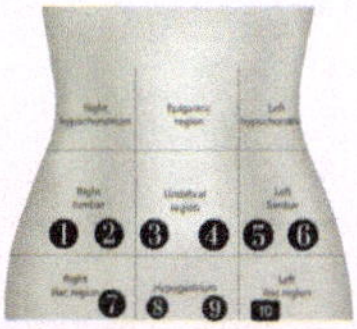

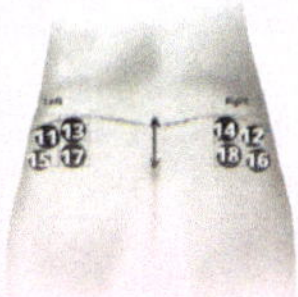

My INJECTIONS

Care Period: ______________ to ______________

Date ____/_____/_____________ Symptoms / Comments: ______________________________

Med Name & Dosage	Route	Site #	Stork Name

Date ____/_____/_____________ Symptoms / Comments: ______________________________

Med Name & Dosage	Route	Site #	Stork Name

Date ____/_____/_____________ Symptoms / Comments: ______________________________

Med Name & Dosage	Route	Site #	Stork Name

Date ____/_____/_____________ Symptoms / Comments: ______________________________

Med Name & Dosage	Route	Site #	Stork Name

Date ____/_____/_____________ Symptoms / Comments: ______________________________

Med Name & Dosage	Route	Site #	Stork Name

Date ____/_____/_____________ Symptoms / Comments: ______________________________

Med Name & Dosage	Route	Site #	Stork Name

Date ____/_____/_____________ Symptoms / Comments: ______________________________

Med Name & Dosage	Route	Site #	Stork Name

Date ____/_____/_____________ Symptoms / Comments: ______________________________

Med Name & Dosage	Route	Site #	Stork Name

INJECTION SITES:

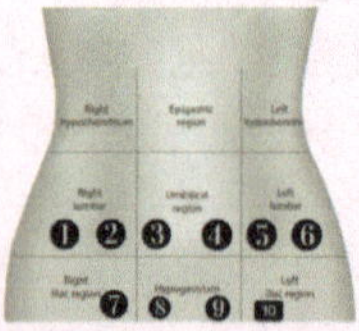

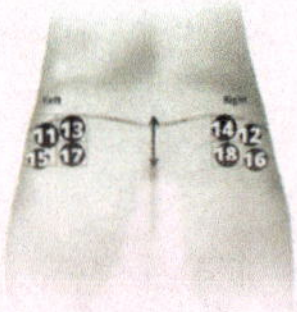

My INJECTIONS

Care Period: ______________ to ______________

Date ____ /____ /__________ Symptoms / Comments: ______________________

Med Name & Dosage	Route	Site #	Stork Name

Date ____ /____ /__________ Symptoms / Comments: ______________________

Med Name & Dosage	Route	Site #	Stork Name

Date ____ /____ /__________ Symptoms / Comments: ______________________

Med Name & Dosage	Route	Site #	Stork Name

Date ____ /____ /__________ Symptoms / Comments: ______________________

Med Name & Dosage	Route	Site #	Stork Name

Date ____ /____ /__________ Symptoms / Comments: ______________________

Med Name & Dosage	Route	Site #	Stork Name

Date ____ /____ /__________ Symptoms / Comments: ______________________

Med Name & Dosage	Route	Site #	Stork Name

Date ____ /____ /__________ Symptoms / Comments: ______________________

Med Name & Dosage	Route	Site #	Stork Name

Date ____ /____ /__________ Symptoms / Comments: ______________________

Med Name & Dosage	Route	Site #	Stork Name

INJECTION SITES:

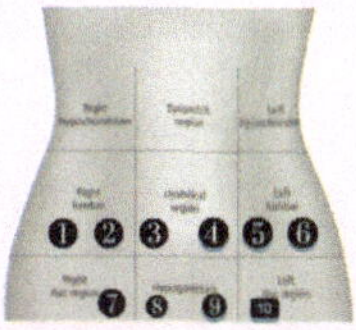

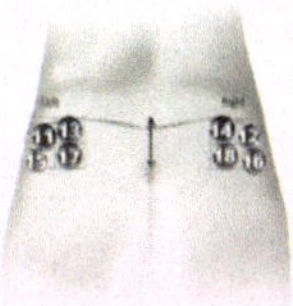

My NOTES

Date:

My EMBRYOS

Date: _______ /_______ /____________ Follicles Retrieved: ______________________________________

Mature Follicles _________________________ ICSI/PICSI: ____________________________________

Day	1	3	5	6	Blastocysts	Frozen	PGS Normal	PGS Abnormal
Qty								

pgt / pgs / pgd Results

Embryo #	Morphology	Embryo Result	Grade	Sex	Notes

Retrieval Day Check In

Doctor Name: ______________________________ Location: ____

My NOTES

Date:

"CLients Corner"

Thank you
for always being
my hype girl am encouraging
me to keep doing the dang thing!
You are a wonderful person with
a huge heart!

Love, ♥

My CYCLE # ________

Start Date:

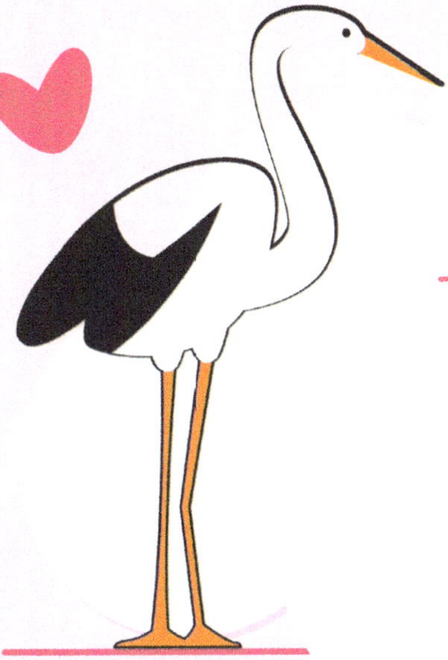

Trust the Process

My MED CHECKS

Date of *Initial* Med Check: ____________________ Notes: ____

Date	Med Name & Dosage	# of doses remaining	Earliest Reorder date	Storage after opening

Date	Med Name & Dosage	# of doses remaining	Earliest Reorder date	Storage after opening

Date	Med Name & Dosage	# of doses remaining	Earliest Reorder date	Storage after opening

Date	Med Name & Dosage	# of doses remaining	Earliest Reorder date	Storage after opening

Date	Med Name & Dosage	# of doses remaining	Earliest Reorder date	Storage after opening

Date	Med Name & Dosage	# of doses remaining	Earliest Reorder date	Storage after opening

Date	Med Name & Dosage	# of doses remaining	Earliest Reorder date	Storage after opening

★ Note: Meds generally expire within 28 days of piercing vial or by expiration date, whichever is sooner.

My IVF SCHEDULE

SUPPRESION CHECK:	STIM DAY 1	STIM DAY 2	STIM DAY 3	STIM DAY 4
BASELINE ULTRASOUND & BLOOD TEST	Start Stim Meds			
Period day 1	**PM Stim Meds:** Gonal-F / FSH / Menopur / MiniHCG / Omnitrope			
	AM Meds : If on Lupron protocol, continue Lupron AM			

STIM DAY 5	STIM DAY 6	STIM DAY 7	STIM DAY 8	STIM DAY 9
Day 5 or 6 1st AM Monitoring Appt.				Day 9 Appt.
PM Stim Meds: Gonal-F / FSH / Menopur / MiniHCG / Omnitrope				
AM Cetrotide / Ganirelix only once instructed to start *OR* continue Lupron				

STIM DAY 10	STIM DAY 11	STIM DAY 12	STIM DAY 13	STIM DAY 14
PM Stim Meds: Gonal-F / FSH / Menopur / MiniHCG / Omnitrope				
AM Cetrotide / Ganirelix *OR* continue Lupron				
90% chance of HCG PM Trigger			10% chance of HCG PM Trigger	
			90% chance of AM Egg Retrieval	

10% chance of AM Egg Retrieval

Fresh Embryo Transfer: 3 to 5 days post - Egg Retrieval *OR*
Frozen Embryo BIOPSY: 5 to 7 Days post-Egg Retrieval

IMPORTANT DATES / TIMES

(Email CNS office ASAP if outside your time window)

Clinic Monitoring Appointments

Day 5 / 6: ____ /____ /________ Time: ______
Day 9: ____ /____ /________ Time: ______
Day ___: ____ /____ /________ Time: ______
Day ___: ____ /____ /________ Time: ______
Day ___: ____ /____ /________ Time: ______
Day ___: ____ /____ /________ Time: ______

1st Cetrotide / Ganirelix shot

Date: ____ /____ /________ Time: ______PM

Email CNS office ASAP with details!

Trigger Shot
Date: ____ /____ /________ Time: ______PM

My APPOINTMENTS

DATE & TIME: ______________________ ______________________

APPOINTMENT TYPE: ______________________

- ❒ CONSULTATION
- ❒ CYCLE MONITORING
- ❒ EGG RETRIEVAL
- ❒ LABS
- ❒ PROCEDURE(S)
- ❒ ULTRASOUND
- ❒ FET/TRANSFER
- ❒ OTHER

QUESTIONS/CONCERNS BEFORE APPT/TOPICS DISCUSSED WITH CNS STORK:

INSTRUCTIONS/FOLLOW-UP/NOTES/EMAIL CNS OFFICE

BLOOD TEST

Date	Blood test type	Expected Normal Range(s)	My Results

FOLLICLE GROWTH

Date	Lining Thickness (mm)	Left Ovary		Right Ovary	
		#	Size	#	Size

My APPOINTMENTS

DATE & TIME: ______________________ ______________________

APPOINTMENT TYPE: ______________________

- ❐ CONSULTATION
- ❐ CYCLE MONITORING
- ❐ EGG RETRIEVAL
- ❐ LABS
- ❐ PROCEDURE(S)
- ❐ ULTRASOUND
- ❐ FET/TRANSFER
- ❐ OTHER

QUESTIONS/CONCERNS BEFORE APPT/TOPICS DISCUSSED WITH CNS STORK:

____

____

INSTRUCTIONS/FOLLOW-UP/NOTES/EMAIL CNS OFFICE

____

____

BLOOD TEST

Date	Blood test type	Expected Normal Range(s)	My Results

FOLLICLE GROWTH

Date	Lining Thickness (mm)	Left Ovary		Right Ovary	
		#	Size	#	Size

My APPOINTMENTS

DATE & TIME: ______________________ ______________________

APPOINTMENT TYPE: ______________________

☐ CONSULTATION	☐ CYCLE MONITORING	☐ EGG RETRIEVAL	☐ LABS
☐ PROCEDURE(S)	☐ ULTRASOUND	☐ FET/TRANSFER	☐ OTHER

QUESTIONS/CONCERNS BEFORE APPT/TOPICS DISCUSSED WITH CNS STORK:

INSTRUCTIONS/FOLLOW-UP/NOTES/EMAIL CNS OFFICE

BLOOD TEST

Date	Blood test type	Expected Normal Range(s)	My Results

FOLLICLE GROWTH

Date	Lining Thickness (mm)	Left Ovary		Right Ovary	
		#	Size	#	Size

My APPOINTMENTS

DATE & TIME: ______________________ ______________________

APPOINTMENT TYPE: ______________________________________

- ❒ CONSULTATION
- ❒ CYCLE MONITORING
- ❒ EGG RETRIEVAL
- ❒ LABS
- ❒ PROCEDURE(S)
- ❒ ULTRASOUND
- ❒ FET/TRANSFER
- ❒ OTHER

QUESTIONS/CONCERNS BEFORE APPT/TOPICS DISCUSSED WITH CNS STORK:

INSTRUCTIONS/FOLLOW-UP/NOTES/EMAIL CNS OFFICE

BLOOD TEST

Date	Blood test type	Expected Normal Range(s)	My Results

FOLLICLE GROWTH

Date	Lining Thickness (mm)	Left Ovary		Right Ovary	
		#	Size	#	Size

My APPOINTMENTS

DATE & TIME: ________________________ ________________________

APPOINTMENT TYPE: ____

- ❑ CONSULTATION
- ❑ CYCLE MONITORING
- ❑ EGG RETRIEVAL
- ❑ LABS
- ❑ PROCEDURE(S)
- ❑ ULTRASOUND
- ❑ FET/TRANSFER
- ❑ OTHER

QUESTIONS/CONCERNS BEFORE APPT/TOPICS DISCUSSED WITH CNS STORK:

INSTRUCTIONS/FOLLOW-UP/NOTES/EMAIL CNS OFFICE

BLOOD TEST

Date	Blood test type	Expected Normal Range(s)	My Results

FOLLICLE GROWTH

Date	Lining Thickness (mm)	Left Ovary		Right Ovary	
		#	Size	#	Size

My APPOINTMENTS

DATE & TIME: ______________________ ______________________

APPOINTMENT TYPE: ______________________

- ❒ CONSULTATION
- ❒ CYCLE MONITORING
- ❒ EGG RETRIEVAL
- ❒ LABS
- ❒ PROCEDURE(S)
- ❒ ULTRASOUND
- ❒ FET/TRANSFER
- ❒ OTHER

QUESTIONS/CONCERNS BEFORE APPT/TOPICS DISCUSSED WITH CNS STORK:

INSTRUCTIONS/FOLLOW-UP/NOTES/EMAIL CNS OFFICE

BLOOD TEST

Date	Blood test type	Expected Normal Range(s)	My Results

FOLLICLE GROWTH

Date	Lining Thickness (mm)	Left Ovary		Right Ovary	
		#	Size	#	Size

My INJECTIONS

Care Period: ________________ to ________________

Date ____ /_____ /_____________ Symptoms / Comments: ______________________________

Med Name & Dosage	Route	Site #	Stork Name

Date ____ /_____ /_____________ Symptoms / Comments: ______________________________

Med Name & Dosage	Route	Site #	Stork Name

Date ____ /_____ /_____________ Symptoms / Comments: ______________________________

Med Name & Dosage	Route	Site #	Stork Name

Date ____ /_____ /_____________ Symptoms / Comments: ______________________________

Med Name & Dosage	Route	Site #	Stork Name

Date ____ /_____ /_____________ Symptoms / Comments: ______________________________

Med Name & Dosage	Route	Site #	Stork Name

Date ____ /_____ /_____________ Symptoms / Comments: ______________________________

Med Name & Dosage	Route	Site #	Stork Name

Date ____ /_____ /_____________ Symptoms / Comments: ______________________________

Med Name & Dosage	Route	Site #	Stork Name

Date ____ /_____ /_____________ Symptoms / Comments: ______________________________

Med Name & Dosage	Route	Site #	Stork Name

INJECTION SITES:

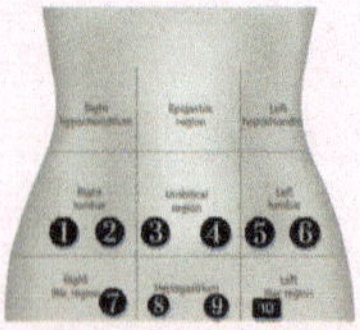

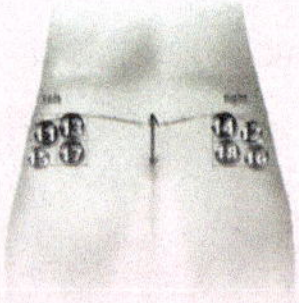

My INJECTIONS

Care Period: ______________ to ______________

Date ____ /_____ /____________ Symptoms / Comments: ____________________________

Med Name & Dosage	Route	Site #	Stork Name

Date ____ /_____ /____________ Symptoms / Comments: ____________________________

Med Name & Dosage	Route	Site #	Stork Name

Date ____ /_____ /____________ Symptoms / Comments: ____________________________

Med Name & Dosage	Route	Site #	Stork Name

Date ____ /_____ /____________ Symptoms / Comments: ____________________________

Med Name & Dosage	Route	Site #	Stork Name

Date ____ /_____ /____________ Symptoms / Comments: ____________________________

Med Name & Dosage	Route	Site #	Stork Name

Date ____ /_____ /____________ Symptoms / Comments: ____________________________

Med Name & Dosage	Route	Site #	Stork Name

Date ____ /_____ /____________ Symptoms / Comments: ____________________________

Med Name & Dosage	Route	Site #	Stork Name

Date ____ /_____ /____________ Symptoms / Comments: ____________________________

Med Name & Dosage	Route	Site #	Stork Name

INJECTION SITES:

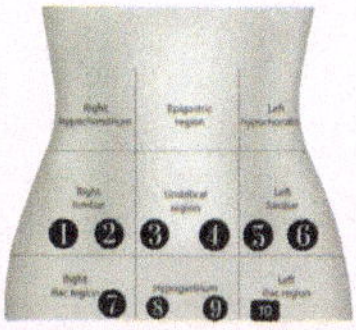

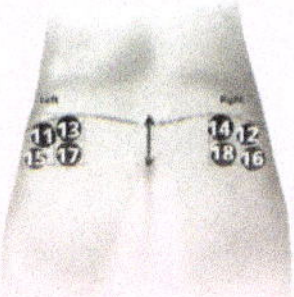

My INJECTIONS

Care Period: ______________ **to** ______________

Date ____/_____/____________ Symptoms / Comments: ______________________________

Med Name & Dosage	Route	Site #	Stork Name

Date ____/_____/____________ Symptoms / Comments: ______________________________

Med Name & Dosage	Route	Site #	Stork Name

Date ____/_____/____________ Symptoms / Comments: ______________________________

Med Name & Dosage	Route	Site #	Stork Name

Date ____/_____/____________ Symptoms / Comments: ______________________________

Med Name & Dosage	Route	Site #	Stork Name

Date ____/_____/____________ Symptoms / Comments: ______________________________

Med Name & Dosage	Route	Site #	Stork Name

Date ____/_____/____________ Symptoms / Comments: ______________________________

Med Name & Dosage	Route	Site #	Stork Name

Date ____/_____/____________ Symptoms / Comments: ______________________________

Med Name & Dosage	Route	Site #	Stork Name

Date ____/_____/____________ Symptoms / Comments: ______________________________

Med Name & Dosage	Route	Site #	Stork Name

INJECTION SITES:

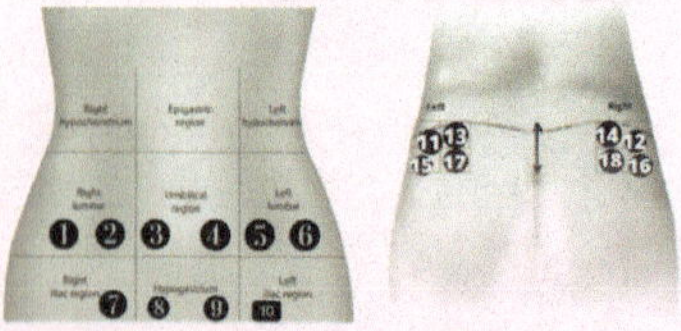

My INJECTIONS

Care Period: ________________ to ________________

Date ____ /_____ /____________ Symptoms / Comments: ______________________________

Med Name & Dosage	Route	Site #	Stork Name

Date ____ /_____ /____________ Symptoms / Comments: ______________________________

Med Name & Dosage	Route	Site #	Stork Name

Date ____ /_____ /____________ Symptoms / Comments: ______________________________

Med Name & Dosage	Route	Site #	Stork Name

Date ____ /_____ /____________ Symptoms / Comments: ______________________________

Med Name & Dosage	Route	Site #	Stork Name

Date ____ /_____ /____________ Symptoms / Comments: ______________________________

Med Name & Dosage	Route	Site #	Stork Name

Date ____ /_____ /____________ Symptoms / Comments: ______________________________

Med Name & Dosage	Route	Site #	Stork Name

Date ____ /_____ /____________ Symptoms / Comments: ______________________________

Med Name & Dosage	Route	Site #	Stork Name

Date ____ /_____ /____________ Symptoms / Comments: ______________________________

Med Name & Dosage	Route	Site #	Stork Name

INJECTION SITES:

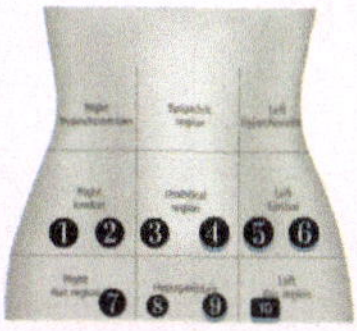

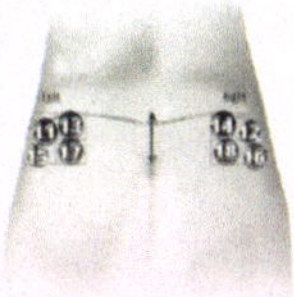

My INJECTIONS

Care Period: ______________ to ______________

Date ____ /_____ /____________ Symptoms / Comments: ______________________________

Med Name & Dosage	Route	Site #	Stork Name

Date ____ /_____ /____________ Symptoms / Comments: ______________________________

Med Name & Dosage	Route	Site #	Stork Name

Date ____ /_____ /____________ Symptoms / Comments: ______________________________

Med Name & Dosage	Route	Site #	Stork Name

Date ____ /_____ /____________ Symptoms / Comments: ______________________________

Med Name & Dosage	Route	Site #	Stork Name

Date ____ /_____ /____________ Symptoms / Comments: ______________________________

Med Name & Dosage	Route	Site #	Stork Name

Date ____ /_____ /____________ Symptoms / Comments: ______________________________

Med Name & Dosage	Route	Site #	Stork Name

Date ____ /_____ /____________ Symptoms / Comments: ______________________________

Med Name & Dosage	Route	Site #	Stork Name

Date ____ /_____ /____________ Symptoms / Comments: ______________________________

Med Name & Dosage	Route	Site #	Stork Name

INJECTION SITES:

____

____

____

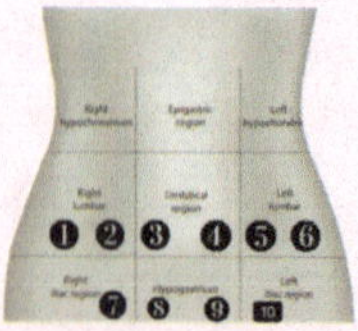

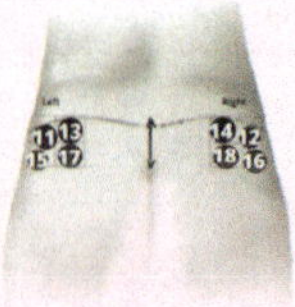

My INJECTIONS

Care Period: ______________ to ______________

Date ____ /_____ /_____________ Symptoms / Comments: ______________________________

Med Name & Dosage	Route	Site #	Stork Name

Date ____ /_____ /_____________ Symptoms / Comments: ______________________________

Med Name & Dosage	Route	Site #	Stork Name

Date ____ /_____ /_____________ Symptoms / Comments: ______________________________

Med Name & Dosage	Route	Site #	Stork Name

Date ____ /_____ /_____________ Symptoms / Comments: ______________________________

Med Name & Dosage	Route	Site #	Stork Name

Date ____ /_____ /_____________ Symptoms / Comments: ______________________________

Med Name & Dosage	Route	Site #	Stork Name

Date ____ /_____ /_____________ Symptoms / Comments: ______________________________

Med Name & Dosage	Route	Site #	Stork Name

Date ____ /_____ /_____________ Symptoms / Comments: ______________________________

Med Name & Dosage	Route	Site #	Stork Name

Date ____ /_____ /_____________ Symptoms / Comments: ______________________________

Med Name & Dosage	Route	Site #	Stork Name

INJECTION SITES:

____

____

____

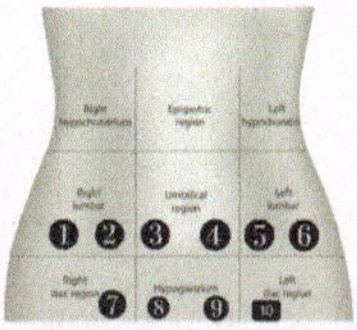

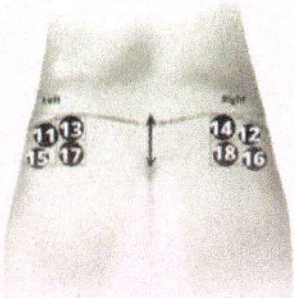

My NOTES

Date:

My EMBRYOS

Date: ______ /______ /__________ Follicles Retrieved: ______________________________

Mature Follicles ____________________ ICSI/PICSI: ______________________________

Day	1	3	5	6	Blastocysts	Frozen	PGS Normal	PGS Abnormal
Qty								

pgt / pgs / pgd Results

Embryo #	Morphology	Embryo Result	Grade	Sex	Notes

Retrieval Day Check In

Doctor Name: ______________________ Location: ______________________________

My NOTES

Date:

"Clients Corner"

Dearest ,

Thank you so much for being a part of our story. I believe in Divine appointments, and you entering our lives, feels like a God send! ♡ Ü Thank you for sharing your beautiful, radiant light with us! We are inspired by you, and cherish your presence in our lives, and this world. From the moment God gave me your name in a dream, prior to us →

"CLients Corner"

connecting with you via
the nursing service, you came
in the dream accompanied
by my Spiritual family, and
I knew you would feel like
family. I pray abundant
blessings over your life and
sweet family, and hope we
can all stay connected.
Thank you doesn't capture my
heart, but I pray you know
how deep my gratitude is for you.
With love,

My CYCLE # ________

Start Date:

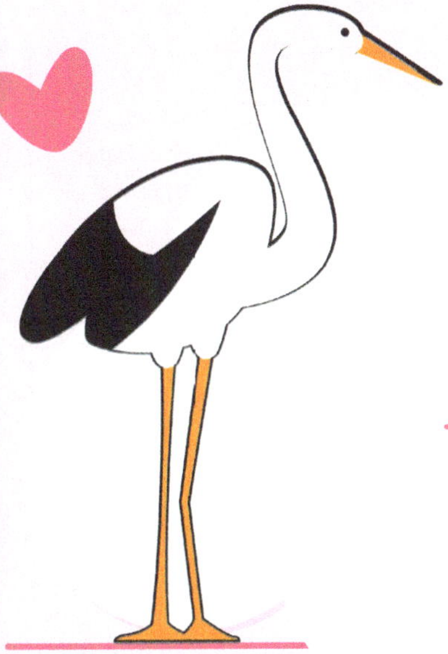

Positive Thoughts

My MED CHECKS

Date of *Initial* Med Check: ____________________ Notes: ____

Date	Med Name & Dosage	# of doses remaining	Earliest Reorder date	Storage after opening

Date	Med Name & Dosage	# of doses remaining	Earliest Reorder date	Storage after opening

Date	Med Name & Dosage	# of doses remaining	Earliest Reorder date	Storage after opening

Date	Med Name & Dosage	# of doses remaining	Earliest Reorder date	Storage after opening

Date	Med Name & Dosage	# of doses remaining	Earliest Reorder date	Storage after opening

Date	Med Name & Dosage	# of doses remaining	Earliest Reorder date	Storage after opening

Date	Med Name & Dosage	# of doses remaining	Earliest Reorder date	Storage after opening

★ Note: Meds generally expire within 28 days of piercing vial or by expiration date, whichever is sooner.

My IVF SCHEDULE

SUPPRESION CHECK:	STIM DAY 1	STIM DAY 2	STIM DAY 3	STIM DAY 4
BASELINE ULTRASOUND & BLOOD TEST	Start Stim Meds			
Period day 1	PM Stim Meds: Gonal-F / FSH / Menopur / MiniHCG / Omnitrope			
	AM Meds : If on Lupron protocol, continue Lupron AM			

STIM DAY 5	STIM DAY 6	STIM DAY 7	STIM DAY 8	STIM DAY 9
Day 5 or 6 1st AM Monitoring Appt.				Day 9 Appt.
PM Stim Meds: Gonal-F / FSH / Menopur / MiniHCG / Omnitrope				
AM Cetrotide / Ganirelix only once instructed to start *OR* continue Lupron				

STIM DAY 10	STIM DAY 11	STIM DAY 12	STIM DAY 13	STIM DAY 14
PM Stim Meds: Gonal-F / FSH / Menopur / MiniHCG / Omnitrope				
AM Cetrotide / Ganirelix *OR* continue Lupron				
90% chance of HCG PM Trigger			10% chance of HCG PM Trigger	
		90% chance of AM Egg Retrieval		

10% chance of AM Egg Retrieval

Fresh Embryo Transfer: 3 to 5 days post - Egg Retrieval *OR*
Frozen Embryo BIOPSY: 5 to 7 Days post-Egg Retrieval

IMPORTANT DATES / TIMES

(Email CNS office ASAP if outside your time window)

Clinic Monitoring Appointments

Day 5 / 6: ____ /____ /_________ Time: ______
Day 9: ____ /____ /_________ Time: ______
Day ___: ____ /____ /_________ Time: ______
Day ___: ____ /____ /_________ Time: ______
Day ___: ____ /____ /_________ Time: ______
Day ___: ____ /____ /_________ Time: ______

1st Cetrotide / Ganirelix shot

Date: ____ /____ /_________ Time: ______PM

Email CNS office ASAP with details!

Trigger Shot

Date: ____ /____ /_________ Time: ______PM

My APPOINTMENTS

DATE & TIME: ______________________ ______________________

APPOINTMENT TYPE: ______________________

☐ CONSULTATION	☐ CYCLE MONITORING	☐ EGG RETRIEVAL	☐ LABS
☐ PROCEDURE(S)	☐ ULTRASOUND	☐ FET/TRANSFER	☐ OTHER

QUESTIONS/CONCERNS BEFORE APPT/TOPICS DISCUSSED WITH CNS STORK:

INSTRUCTIONS/FOLLOW-UP/NOTES/EMAIL CNS OFFICE

BLOOD TEST

Date	Blood test type	Expected Normal Range(s)	My Results

FOLLICLE GROWTH

Date	Lining Thickness (mm)	Left Ovary		Right Ovary	
		#	Size	#	Size

My APPOINTMENTS

DATE & TIME: ______________________ ______________________

APPOINTMENT TYPE: ______________________

- ❐ CONSULTATION
- ❐ CYCLE MONITORING
- ❐ EGG RETRIEVAL
- ❐ LABS
- ❐ PROCEDURE(S)
- ❐ ULTRASOUND
- ❐ FET/TRANSFER
- ❐ OTHER

QUESTIONS/CONCERNS BEFORE APPT/TOPICS DISCUSSED WITH CNS STORK:

INSTRUCTIONS/FOLLOW-UP/NOTES/EMAIL CNS OFFICE

BLOOD TEST

Date	Blood test type	Expected Normal Range(s)	My Results

FOLLICLE GROWTH

Date	Lining Thickness (mm)	Left Ovary		Right Ovary	
		#	Size	#	Size

My APPOINTMENTS

DATE & TIME: ______________________ ______________________

APPOINTMENT TYPE: ______________________

❒ CONSULTATION	❒ CYCLE MONITORING	❒ EGG RETRIEVAL	❒ LABS
❒ PROCEDURE(S)	❒ ULTRASOUND	❒ FET/TRANSFER	❒ OTHER

QUESTIONS/CONCERNS BEFORE APPT/TOPICS DISCUSSED WITH CNS STORK:

INSTRUCTIONS/FOLLOW-UP/NOTES/EMAIL CNS OFFICE

BLOOD TEST

Date	Blood test type	Expected Normal Range(s)	My Results

FOLLICLE GROWTH

Date	Lining Thickness (mm)	Left Ovary		Right Ovary	
		#	Size	#	Size

My APPOINTMENTS

DATE & TIME: ______________________ ______________________

APPOINTMENT TYPE: ______________________

- ❒ CONSULTATION
- ❒ CYCLE MONITORING
- ❒ EGG RETRIEVAL
- ❒ LABS
- ❒ PROCEDURE(S)
- ❒ ULTRASOUND
- ❒ FET/TRANSFER
- ❒ OTHER

QUESTIONS/CONCERNS BEFORE APPT/TOPICS DISCUSSED WITH CNS STORK:

INSTRUCTIONS/FOLLOW-UP/NOTES/EMAIL CNS OFFICE

BLOOD TEST

Date	Blood test type	Expected Normal Range(s)	My Results

FOLLICLE GROWTH

Date	Lining Thickness (mm)	Left Ovary		Right Ovary	
		#	Size	#	Size

My APPOINTMENTS

DATE & TIME: ______________________ ______________________

APPOINTMENT TYPE: ______________________

❑ CONSULTATION	❑ CYCLE MONITORING	❑ EGG RETRIEVAL	❑ LABS
❑ PROCEDURE(S)	❑ ULTRASOUND	❑ FET/TRANSFER	❑ OTHER

QUESTIONS/CONCERNS BEFORE APPT/TOPICS DISCUSSED WITH CNS STORK:

INSTRUCTIONS/FOLLOW-UP/NOTES/EMAIL CNS OFFICE

BLOOD TEST

Date	Blood test type	Expected Normal Range(s)	My Results

FOLLICLE GROWTH

Date	Lining Thickness (mm)	Left Ovary		Right Ovary	
		#	Size	#	Size

My APPOINTMENTS

DATE & TIME: ______________________ ______________________

APPOINTMENT TYPE: ______________________

- [ ] CONSULTATION
- [ ] CYCLE MONITORING
- [ ] EGG RETRIEVAL
- [ ] LABS
- [ ] PROCEDURE(S)
- [ ] ULTRASOUND
- [ ] FET/TRANSFER
- [ ] OTHER

QUESTIONS/CONCERNS BEFORE APPT/TOPICS DISCUSSED WITH CNS STORK:

INSTRUCTIONS/FOLLOW-UP/NOTES/EMAIL CNS OFFICE

BLOOD TEST

Date	Blood test type	Expected Normal Range(s)	My Results

FOLLICLE GROWTH

Date	Lining Thickness (mm)	Left Ovary		Right Ovary	
		#	Size	#	Size

My INJECTIONS

Care Period: ________________ to ________________

Date ____ /_____ /_____________ Symptoms / Comments: ______________________________

Med Name & Dosage	Route	Site #	Stork Name

Date ____ /_____ /_____________ Symptoms / Comments: ______________________________

Med Name & Dosage	Route	Site #	Stork Name

Date ____ /_____ /_____________ Symptoms / Comments: ______________________________

Med Name & Dosage	Route	Site #	Stork Name

Date ____ /_____ /_____________ Symptoms / Comments: ______________________________

Med Name & Dosage	Route	Site #	Stork Name

Date ____ /_____ /_____________ Symptoms / Comments: ______________________________

Med Name & Dosage	Route	Site #	Stork Name

Date ____ /_____ /_____________ Symptoms / Comments: ______________________________

Med Name & Dosage	Route	Site #	Stork Name

Date ____ /_____ /_____________ Symptoms / Comments: ______________________________

Med Name & Dosage	Route	Site #	Stork Name

Date ____ /_____ /_____________ Symptoms / Comments: ______________________________

Med Name & Dosage	Route	Site #	Stork Name

INJECTION SITES:

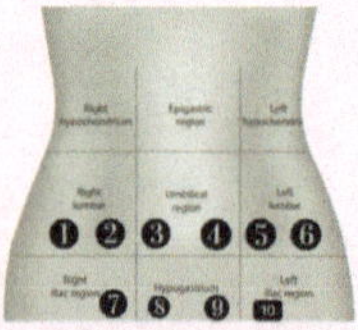

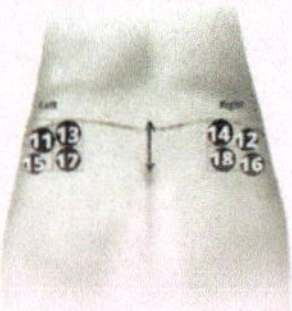

My INJECTIONS

Care Period: ______________ to ______________

Date ____ /_____ /____________ Symptoms / Comments: ______________________

Med Name & Dosage	Route	Site #	Stork Name

Date ____ /_____ /____________ Symptoms / Comments: ______________________

Med Name & Dosage	Route	Site #	Stork Name

Date ____ /_____ /____________ Symptoms / Comments: ______________________

Med Name & Dosage	Route	Site #	Stork Name

Date ____ /_____ /____________ Symptoms / Comments: ______________________

Med Name & Dosage	Route	Site #	Stork Name

Date ____ /_____ /____________ Symptoms / Comments: ______________________

Med Name & Dosage	Route	Site #	Stork Name

Date ____ /_____ /____________ Symptoms / Comments: ______________________

Med Name & Dosage	Route	Site #	Stork Name

Date ____ /_____ /____________ Symptoms / Comments: ______________________

Med Name & Dosage	Route	Site #	Stork Name

Date ____ /_____ /____________ Symptoms / Comments: ______________________

Med Name & Dosage	Route	Site #	Stork Name

INJECTION SITES:

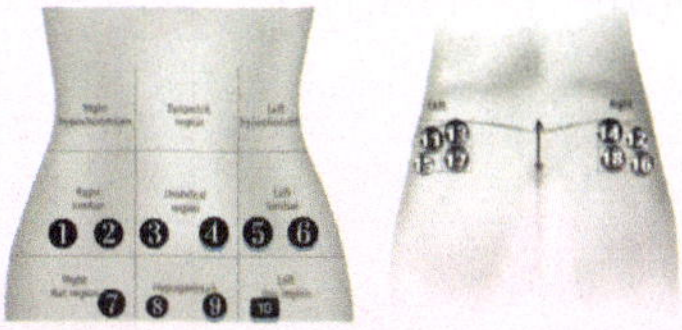

My INJECTIONS

Care Period: ______________ to ______________

Date ____ /_____ /____________ Symptoms / Comments: ______________________________

Med Name & Dosage	Route	Site #	Stork Name

Date ____ /_____ /____________ Symptoms / Comments: ______________________________

Med Name & Dosage	Route	Site #	Stork Name

Date ____ /_____ /____________ Symptoms / Comments: ______________________________

Med Name & Dosage	Route	Site #	Stork Name

Date ____ /_____ /____________ Symptoms / Comments: ______________________________

Med Name & Dosage	Route	Site #	Stork Name

Date ____ /_____ /____________ Symptoms / Comments: ______________________________

Med Name & Dosage	Route	Site #	Stork Name

Date ____ /_____ /____________ Symptoms / Comments: ______________________________

Med Name & Dosage	Route	Site #	Stork Name

Date ____ /_____ /____________ Symptoms / Comments: ______________________________

Med Name & Dosage	Route	Site #	Stork Name

Date ____ /_____ /____________ Symptoms / Comments: ______________________________

Med Name & Dosage	Route	Site #	Stork Name

INJECTION SITES:

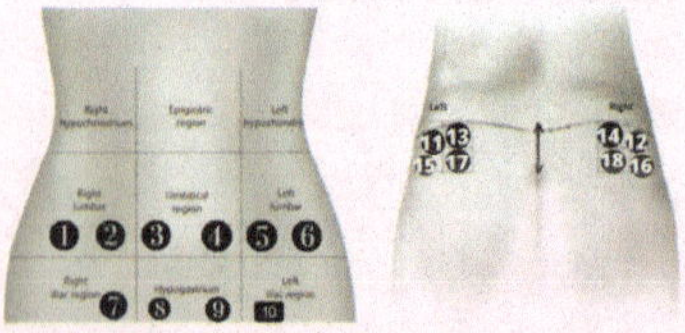

My INJECTIONS

Care Period: ______________ to ______________

Date ____/____/__________ Symptoms / Comments: ______________________________

Med Name & Dosage	Route	Site #	Stork Name

Date ____/____/__________ Symptoms / Comments: ______________________________

Med Name & Dosage	Route	Site #	Stork Name

Date ____/____/__________ Symptoms / Comments: ______________________________

Med Name & Dosage	Route	Site #	Stork Name

Date ____/____/__________ Symptoms / Comments: ______________________________

Med Name & Dosage	Route	Site #	Stork Name

Date ____/____/__________ Symptoms / Comments: ______________________________

Med Name & Dosage	Route	Site #	Stork Name

Date ____/____/__________ Symptoms / Comments: ______________________________

Med Name & Dosage	Route	Site #	Stork Name

Date ____/____/__________ Symptoms / Comments: ______________________________

Med Name & Dosage	Route	Site #	Stork Name

Date ____/____/__________ Symptoms / Comments: ______________________________

Med Name & Dosage	Route	Site #	Stork Name

INJECTION SITES:

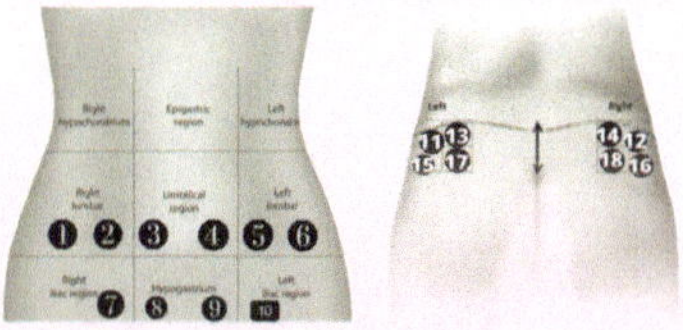

My INJECTIONS

Care Period: ______________ to ______________

Date ____ /_____ /____________ Symptoms / Comments: ______________________________

Med Name & Dosage	Route	Site #	Stork Name

Date ____ /_____ /____________ Symptoms / Comments: ______________________________

Med Name & Dosage	Route	Site #	Stork Name

Date ____ /_____ /____________ Symptoms / Comments: ______________________________

Med Name & Dosage	Route	Site #	Stork Name

Date ____ /_____ /____________ Symptoms / Comments: ______________________________

Med Name & Dosage	Route	Site #	Stork Name

Date ____ /_____ /____________ Symptoms / Comments: ______________________________

Med Name & Dosage	Route	Site #	Stork Name

Date ____ /_____ /____________ Symptoms / Comments: ______________________________

Med Name & Dosage	Route	Site #	Stork Name

Date ____ /_____ /____________ Symptoms / Comments: ______________________________

Med Name & Dosage	Route	Site #	Stork Name

Date ____ /_____ /____________ Symptoms / Comments: ______________________________

Med Name & Dosage	Route	Site #	Stork Name

INJECTION SITES:

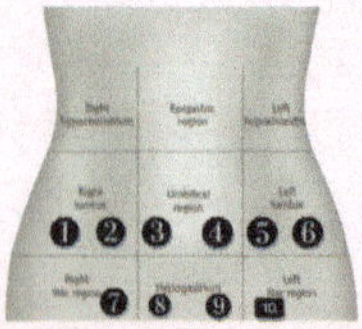

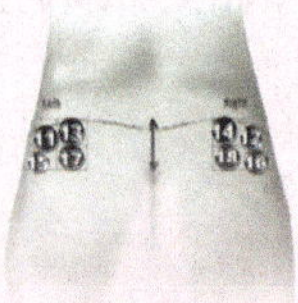

My INJECTIONS

Care Period: ______________ to ______________

Date ____ /_____ /_____________ Symptoms / Comments: ______________________________

Med Name & Dosage	Route	Site #	Stork Name

Date ____ /_____ /_____________ Symptoms / Comments: ______________________________

Med Name & Dosage	Route	Site #	Stork Name

Date ____ /_____ /_____________ Symptoms / Comments: ______________________________

Med Name & Dosage	Route	Site #	Stork Name

Date ____ /_____ /_____________ Symptoms / Comments: ______________________________

Med Name & Dosage	Route	Site #	Stork Name

Date ____ /_____ /_____________ Symptoms / Comments: ______________________________

Med Name & Dosage	Route	Site #	Stork Name

Date ____ /_____ /_____________ Symptoms / Comments: ______________________________

Med Name & Dosage	Route	Site #	Stork Name

Date ____ /_____ /_____________ Symptoms / Comments: ______________________________

Med Name & Dosage	Route	Site #	Stork Name

Date ____ /_____ /_____________ Symptoms / Comments: ______________________________

Med Name & Dosage	Route	Site #	Stork Name

INJECTION SITES:

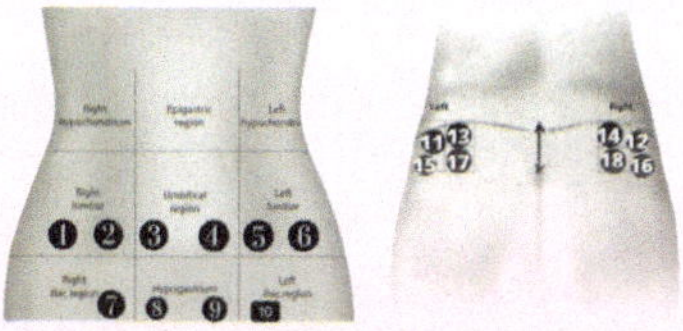

My NOTES

Date:

My EMBRYOS

Date: _______ /_______ /____________ Follicles Retrieved: ______________________________

Mature Follicles ___________________________ ICSI/PICSI: ______________________________

Day	1	3	5	6	Blastocysts	Frozen	PGS Normal	PGS Abnormal
Qty								

pgt / pgs / pgd Results

Embryo #	Morphology	Embryo Result	Grade	Sex	Notes

Retrieval Day Check In

Doctor Name: ______________________________ Location: ______________________________

My NOTES

Date:

My NOTES

Date:

My NOTES

Date:

My NOTES

Date:

Complete
Nurturing
Solutions
Childress Nursing Services

SocioMaternal Home Health

from pre-conception to post-delivery

Made in United States
North Haven, CT
11 November 2026

22095615R10055